THE
UNSPOKEN
WORDS

What Every Health Care Professional Would Love to Say to a Patient and Can't.

M.J. Musgrave

authorHOUSE®

AuthorHouse™
1663 Liberty Drive
Bloomington, IN 47403
www.authorhouse.com
Phone: 1 (800) 839-8640

Published by AuthorHouse 11/18/2017

ISBN: 978-1-5462-1803-6 (sc)
ISBN: 978-1-5462-1804-3 (e)

Print information available on the last page.

This book is printed on acid-free paper.

I always thought I would write a book when I retired from medicine. I have been working in the medical field as a certified nurse practitioner for forty years. I have seen and heard a lot. I started my career providing care in a family practice setting and ended it in an urgent care facility. I also worked in the county health department and occupational health, and I was a director of nursing for a hospital. Over the years, I have had to control what I would love to say and couldn't, as do all medical providers. Our patients are consumers or our customers, and just like a clerk in a store or a waitress, you have to put on your smiley face and aim to please.

All health care providers—including physicians, nurse practitioners, physician assistants, lab techs, radiology techs, nurses, and receptionists—have to watch what they say. If only we could tell patients what they really need to be told.

We go to school a long time to have the ability to differentiate all the possibilities that might cause the symptoms our patients describe. We and our families sacrificed a lot while we went through this training and became good at what we do. Yet since the Internet has arrived, patients think they know what is wrong with them before we even enter the room. They have gotten their degrees from the University of Google and listen to Dr. Google before they do us. They also like to tell us what medicine they want. So I'm starting to think they would be happy if we were like Mexico, where you can walk into a pharmacy and self-medicate. Or maybe we just need to put out vending machines and label them with the different reasons that certain items are taken. When I first started practicing, the patients trusted our judgment and appreciated our knowledge in treating them. But it's not that way anymore. We try to not degrade them when they are wrong, but sometimes they still take it that way.

Over the years, I have also seen many changes in medicine and how we treat different things. The public believes many old wives' tales out there. For example, yellow-green mucous from your nose and lungs doesn't mean you have a bacterial infection. Oh, there was a tendency to treat these symptoms with an antibiotic years ago, but then we got smarter and realized through studies that viral infections cause discolored mucous and that it takes seven to ten days to develop a sinus infection or other bacterial infections. Most of the general public still thinks that, if you have a fever and colored phlegm, you have a bacterial infection and need that antibiotic. That's one reason we are in trouble with resistances to antibiotics.

Sometimes I think that patients are more addicted to antibiotics than they are to narcotics.

I have had patients come in and demand I give them antibiotics. We should say no more often, but because of patients complaining, we give them a prescription for an antibiotic but try to convince them to try the other medication first. Sometimes I think and hope that they tear up the prescription and don't take it.

The other condition associated with myths is poison ivy. People think the blisters that may develop are filled with poison ivy and are contagious when they bust. I've been told they believe they leave it on the sheets, couch, and other materials. I've also been told that if you have chlamydia, a sexually transmitted disease (STD), you can't masturbate for five days.

In the pages that follow, I'll make you aware of some of the things we hear and how we would love to respond. Hopefully I don't offend you if you have made these comments yourself. There are also some comments that don't need responses.

A person came in for insect bites. When the provider told the patient what they were, the response was, "What kind of insect was it?" When the provider said she didn't know, the patient called her a bitch and said, "I'm paying you to know these things." The provider wanted to respond, "Well, sorry. I majored in medicine, not to be an exterminator."

A patient had rib pain. The provider suggested a rib belt but told the patient he needed to remove it every one to two hours to take deep breaths. The patient proceeded to tell the provider he didn't know what the provider was talking about, that the Internet said not to use them anymore because they constricted one's breathing. And the patient left without paying the bill.

A patient came in with her husband. She was eight months pregnant. She had a cold, but when I asked what she was having, she stated they were going to be surprised and didn't know. Her husband responded, "It better be a boy, or I don't want it." He was not joking. He was dead serious. I just looked at him and said, "You better just wish it is healthy and be thankful with whatever sex it is." Creep!

One day a guy came in with a blue spot on his hand, afraid it was something awful like cancer. We had him go into the bathroom and wash his hands, and it came off. Our tax dollars were at work for that visit.

A patient came in for a cold, and while listening to her lungs, I noticed multiple bruises and scratches across her lower back. I asked if she were being abused, and she replied, "No, it is from sexual activity, and I like it that way." I was so dumbfounded that I couldn't respond. All I could say was, "Well then, I won't worry about them."

Everyone came in thinking he or she had allergies to medicines. Even if it were just a GI disturbance, it was an "allergy." Well, here's one that took the cake: a spermicide listed a possible allergic response. The reaction was, "It causes me gallbladder problems." Now I will never understand how something vaginally can hurt your gallbladder.

Another great allergy comment was, "I'm allergic to penicillin, but you don't use that anymore anyway." I thought, "Please don't tell someone with gonorrhea or strep throat that, or we are in big trouble."

Sometimes patients told more than we wanted to hear. One provider once saw a single girl who he diagnosed as being pregnant. After telling the patient, she said, "Well, you know who the father is? It is your next-door neighbor." Like he really wanted to know that his neighbor, who was married with kids, was the father of this baby. It was a long nine months for that provider.

Many came to the office or department telling us which antibiotic they wanted. They stated, "Nothing else works." Obviously we gave them what was indicated even if it weren't what they wanted, and they got mad. We wanted to say, "Don't you want what is appropriate? And who went to medical school, you or me?" This was a vending machine patient.

Then you got the pediatric patient who was not cooperative with parents who were no help. An eleven-year-old patient came in needing two stitches in his hand. It took four people to hold him down, and his mother kept asking if we couldn't just talk to him, as if we were going to convince him to sit still and let me stick him with a needle by talking to him. The parent should've been helping to hold his arm.

A patient came in saying she drank a lot of caffeine and was concerned because she thought her pee smelled like caffeine. I would love for her to bring in a specimen and have her smell it and state, "Oh, wait till you eat a lot of asparagus."

There were so many stupid drug seekers. We had a pregnant woman who was hopping from ER to ER, seeking narcotics. She had different complaints every place she went, but it was always some type of pain. We'd love to say, "You idiot, hurt yourself but not your innocent child." But obviously we said, "No, take Tylenol."

Some were just really strange. Once a female reported that she had an orgasm every time she moved her bowels. I wanted to respond, "Are you on a laxative? Enjoy yourself! What happens when you pee?"

Then they thought they had some strange thing wrong with them. Someone with diarrhea for five days and continued to eat everything—fast foods, roughage, and pizza—said, "I have this parasite in me." I thought, "How stupid are you? If you have diarrhea, you must let the bowel rest and heal, not load it up with junk."

Pain was a whole different story. People came in with various complaints to get pain pills (narcotics). One time this guy came in with a "headache," and when the provider asked him what he took last for his headache, his response was, "What fuckin' does it matter? Just give me something for pain." Obviously he was told to take Motrin and then discharged.

We got sworn at, and people even put their faces in front of ours, trying to intimidate us to get painkillers. We tried to explain that pain meds didn't take care of what was causing the pain and what we were prescribing would. But what we would have loved to say was, "You asshole, you are an addict, and get your crap off the street, not from us."

A patient refused to let the provider touch her because he used hand sanitizer instead of soap. She stated that hand sanitizer lowered your immunity. I thought, "What the hell are you talking about? It's because you didn't use hand sanitizer that you are here."

A person came in complaining of back pain off and on

for years, and she was only fifteen years old. She was five foot three and weighed 311 pounds. She couldn't help it that she weighed 311 pounds. She had a gland problem. I thought, "Yes, it's your salivary glands. Stop taking food to your mouth so often, and your back won't hurt."

A patient came in, stating, "All the glands in my neck are enlarged. I think I have cancer." Obviously not all the glands in her neck were enlarged. She had a viral pharyngitis. If everyone with a few sore lymph nodes thought he or she had cancer, the oncologist couldn't see them all. If someone was worried more about getting a job and working than spending time on the Internet looking up swollen glands, this person wouldn't be on Medicaid and spending the taxpayers' money coming in here.

A four-year-old was seen with his mother present. When they started to leave, the mother said to him, "Grab your personal effects." The child had a stuffed animal with him. I wanted to say, "You are talking to a four-year-old. Just say your toy." Poor kid was being treated like an adult, and he was only four.

A patient came in with a vaginal problem and said, "I have bumps on my crotch." I wanted to say to her, "Please use another term, like genitals, labia, or even down there." Some people were very vulgar.

A patient came in with an injury to a nail done two days ago and had dried blood and dirt on his finger. He didn't even try to clean it off in two days. I looked at it and ordered the nurse to clean it. I wanted to tell him, "You could have at least washed it off and tried to keep it from getting infected. Soap and water are cheap and go a long way to prevent a wound from getting worse. Do not just expect an antibiotic to do it."

In the same type of situation, a child came in due to stepping on a nail the day before. His feet on the bottom were extremely dirty. I just shook my head, but I wanted to say, "I wouldn't even let my child go to bed that dirty, let alone not clean the wound."

Then of course we heard this a lot, "I need an antibiotic." We all wanted to say, "Why did I go to school so long to learn what I did when you can just tell me how to treat you?"

In another pain situation, a patient came in stating," I am having [elective] surgery in one week. Can I have a shot of Dilaudid?" We wanted to say, "Hell no."

Then there were the ones who came in five minutes before we closed and had been sick for three days. We wanted to ask, "Where have you been for the last twelve hours that we have been open?"

A patient had a concern about a possible STD. I asked if she had more than one sexual partner in the last month. She replied, "Yes, ten to twelve." I wanted to ask, "Are you running a whorehouse? You could make some good money."

There were many old wives' tales about poison ivy and many comments from patients. One was, "I think I inhaled it because I have it on my face and neck. I wanted to reply,"

No, do you think you might have come in contact with it and touched your face?"

Some people really blew things out of proportion. One had a small pimple in front of her ear. She stated, "I think the infection has spread to my teeth and into my throat and my ear." I wanted to say, "Suck it up. It's just a pimple."

Some people had a very low pain threshold but would swear that theirs was very high. An adult with a minor ear infection stated, "It hurts so bad. I can't stand it, and I have a high pain threshold." I wanted to say, "Suck it up. If you were a kid, you wouldn't be complaining at all." This same thing happened if an adult had a fever of a hundred degrees. He or she thought he or she was dying, and a child would be running around the room, acting just fine. People changed when they grew up.

A patient had stubbed her toe, and we wanted to splint it or tape it so she didn't bump it. she said, "Oh, you can't. I can't stand things between my toes." Yet she was wearing flip-flops. I said, "But your shoes are between your toes." And she said, "Oh, that's different."

Some things were just not worth arguing about. I just shook my head and said, "Well, good luck because that is all we can do."

I loved the patients who came in for narcotics and acted like they couldn't say the name of the drug and struggled with Vicodin or hydrocodone. I wanted to say, "Oh, you mean hydrochlorothiazide (a water pill), Vioxx (an arthritis pill), or even Viagra." They said, "No, that's not it." Then I said, "I have no idea, and I'm going to give you an anti-inflammatory." I really wanted to say, "You asshole, go get your drugs somewhere else."

I had one guy who came in and said, "If you don't give me my Xanax, I'm going to have a seizure from stress and hit someone and kill them." My wishful response would have been, "Hey, dude, I'm not the one who is screwed up and didn't get another prescription before I ran out."

We got some really strange workman's comp complaints too. One said she snuffed (sucked up nasal secretions) and strained her neck at work, and she was literally filing workman's comp. I wanted to say on the report, "This is an idiot. What the hell is she thinking?"

Patients didn't like to get on the scales. Who does? One came in for an eye infection and refused to get on the scale. She stated, "What does my eye have to do with my weight?" I would love to say, "Look, stupid. Put your big ass on the scale and get into the room."

Let's talk about chronic illness. This patient said, "I've had bronchitis since I've been thirteen." She was twenty-eight. She reported she had been sick for eighteen hours. I wanted to respond, "What the hell do you want me to do because I'm not going to argue with you? I can't handle this discussion today." Or I pondered saying, "That's too bad. You should be a case study. Let me refer you to a pulmonologist. I can't help you since I'm not qualified to handle such a case."

I had a patient who had some mental handicaps and came in stating she hadn't had a menses for five months. She stated, "It feels like bubbles in my stomach, and something is kicking me in my stomach. I was on birth control, but I stopped it." My desired response was, "You can't even take care of yourself. You shouldn't have a child. Get sterilized." Thank God she wasn't pregnant.

A patient came in reporting nausea and vomiting. He stated, "I had chili yesterday to see if it would help, but it didn't." I wanted to say, "You are an idiot. Why would you try chili when you have vomiting and stomach pains?"

Then we would deal with different cultures and their beliefs. I had a young woman come in with her husband. It was their custom that, after they got married and had intercourse, they must wear red bracelets from their elbow to their wrist for one year. The problem was that she came in with a sprained wrist. I couldn't examine her wrist, and she would not take them off. Then I told her I could not get an x-ray or even wrap it in an Ace wrap. Based on history, it was probably sprained, not fractured, so I put her in a brace. But I had to put it over the bracelets. Sometimes people weren't even cooperative so we could treat them properly. And if they didn't get better, guess whose fault it was? Not theirs.

Patients came in believing all kinds of things, and I wasn't sure where they got their information. A patient stated when I entered the room, "I get sick all the time because I have Factor V Leiden." Factor V Leiden is a clotting problem that makes the person clot easily. It doesn't have anything to do with illness. I wanted to state, "Oh, they changed it. When I went to school, that was a defect in the blood that makes you clot, not get sick. Thanks for letting me know that."

Some patients were so descriptive of their symptoms. One commented, "I yawned, and my tonsil busted open." Gee, if that would happen, we wouldn't have to drain tonsillar abscesses. What a great new technique.

Some descriptions just didn't make sense. A mother brought in a five-month-old, stating he had a cough and was acting fatigued. I thought, "How does a five-month-old act fatigued? Maybe sleeping more, but a five-month-old does not sit around and act tired."

Sometimes the elderly patients really described things differently. An eighty-two-year-old woman said, "I have two bugs under my skin biting me. When you get older, your bladder moves around in your abdomen." I wanted to ask, "Are you sure there isn't three or four bugs, just two?" Her thoughts were so far from reality that it wasn't worth me trying to teach her or explain anything, so I didn't waste my breath.

One time I asked a patient if he could explain to me how his ears felt. His response was, "They feel like shit." I calmly replied, "Can you give me more details?"

Then there were always video descriptions and some with sound effects. I had a girl come in for a hemorrhoid and wanted me to watch a video of what it looked like. Her boyfriend had taken it. She proceeded to show it to me, and they had recorded music with it. I wanted to ask, "Are you planning on using this for YouTube?"

When I was working the prenatal clinic, I would have teenage girls come in together. One of them would be pregnant, and the other one would say, "Wait till you have your second kid. You get a lot more money." Boy, what a goal for our young population.

One major problem has always been the fact that a minor can come in and get treated for STDs or get put on birth control, and we aren't allowed to tell the parents. The parents pay the bill and want to know what the visit was for, and we can't reveal that information. They get mad at us, and I want to say, "If you had a better relationship with your child, he or she would tell you."

We had patients go through our drawers in the examining rooms and take things. We had to remove all our dressings, tape, Band-Aids, and so forth. We couldn't even stop thieves.

A thirteen-year-old came in with chronic back pain. Her weight was 250 pounds. I couldn't tell her that it was due to her weight or tell her she was obese because it might lower her self-esteem. Parents were concerned about that. I thought, "What the hell. Be concerned about her physical health, and you'll help her mental health. Someone who is thirteen shouldn't have chronic problems that could be prevented."

A patient came in for a foreign body in the vagina, a Bic pen. I wanted to say, "Be careful where you sit."

Someone came into urgent care to have a paper filled out to get a free fishing license because of disability. I thought, "This is urgent care. Give me a break."

A patient came in stating she needed a note to have permission to have water at her work site. She stated, "I have to have water every hour, or I will have to quit my job." There was no reason this person needed that much water, and nothing was causing her to be thirsty. She just didn't want to work. I gave her a note to have bottled water, and she was mad I gave her the note. I couldn't win!

Parents could be crazy. A ten-year-old girl came in with her mother. Both the physician and I checked her and told the mother out loud in front of the girl what we thought was wrong. She had contact dermatitis. Before I discharged them, the mother wanted me to go over again with the girl what I thought was wrong and tell her, "Someone cares about you and is trying to take care of your problem." I did what she asked, but it was like, "You have to be kidding me!"

A patient told me that you could clean your sinuses by putting peroxide in your ear. I showed him a drawing of the anatomy of the ear canal and the sinuses and said there was no connection. He still disagreed with me and said it worked. I put peroxide in my ear, and I could breathe just fine. Sometimes it wasn't worth trying to teach someone something that he or she would never understand.

A patient came in saying, "I think I have anal herpes, type one. I had rectal sex four years ago, and my rectum is sore now." I wanted to say, "Well, if you have type one herpes, then someone has been licking your ass." Oral sex causes type one.

A parent brought in a child and stated, "He is allergic to pears. They make his balls itch." I wanted to ask, "When he eats them or rubs them on his balls?"

A woman came in stating, "I have maggots in my vagina because I used mayo as a lubricant and didn't wash it out." I thought, "Well, I'll never eat mayo again. What an idiot!"

A patient came in for suture removal. The nurse put the tray and scissors in the room for the provider to take them out. When the provider entered the room, the instruments were out of their sterile wrappings, and the patient had removed the sutures. He stated, "I got tired of waiting." I wanted to reply, "Boy, I'm sorry. Five to ten minutes is a long time. And guess what? Now we are not responsible for the healing of your wound." What an idiot! The sutures might not have been ready to be removed, but I forgot he went to school to be able to evaluate that.

Some people wanted everything for nothing. A patient had a sprained finger. A nurse took in a splint to apply it. The patient asked, "Do I have to pay for that?" I wanted to say, "No, buddy. We are giving away free splints today."

Another request was for a prescription for acetaminophen and other over-the-counter medicines because welfare would pay for them. We all wanted to say, "Buy it yourself instead of buying cigarettes and beer."

Complaints of pain were always interesting. We rated pain on a scale of one to ten, with ten being the worst. Let me tell you more than 95 percent responded with a ten. One patient stated, "I'm having so much pain (which was musculoskeletal) that I can't stand it." I asked if he tried anything like Motrin, ice, and so on. He responded no. Now wouldn't you think that, if you had that much pain, you would have tried something!

This man came in and told the provider that he had decreased semen production. When getting a thorough history, he reported that he masturbated and ejaculated five times a day on a regular basis. The provider wanted to respond, "Get a new hobby."

A man came in reporting he was taking Premarin, a hormone to make him more feminine, but he got his girlfriend pregnant. He said, "I thought it would make me sterile." I wanted to say, "Now I'm confused, but not as much as you are."

A boyfriend came in with his girlfriend, the patient. She had a yeast infection and wanted to be sure she couldn't give it to him. I wanted to say, "Yes, and it's lethal."

Do you know what Ben Wa balls are? They are a sexual toy, and this guy had an allergic reaction to them. He wore off the chrome plating and stated he took them back for credit. Can you believe that? Patients did the stupidest things.

This patient was seen on a Saturday for back pain. His weight was 332 pounds. He was treated and told to do good stretching exercises. A sheet of exercises was given. He returned on Monday stating he had done some jumping jacks on Sunday, and now his knees hurt. I thought, "Don't do jumping jacks if your back hurts and not until you have lost two hundred pounds."

A woman came in complaining of abdominal pain. The husband wanted to know if she could be pregnant. She had a hysterectomy years ago. I wanted to reply, "Sorry, there is no oven to bake the cake!"

This patient came in stating she had a test done in the emergency department (which included blood work and CT scan) and found to have viral stomach flu. She stated she watched her diet for two days and felt better, but then ate two hot dogs, French fries, and pizza. And now she had nausea and vomiting again and couldn't go to work. I wanted to say, "We just spent several thousands of dollars to diagnose you (which you didn't pay for), and you couldn't stay away from junk food long enough to allow your stomach to heal. You deserve to be sick again."

Here is another example of not having to pay for the visit. This person came in on crutches and a knee brace. He had been seen in the emergency department two days prior and treated for the knee problem, and he would be seeing an orthopedic doctor in two days. He came in urgent care just to get a work note for the next two days. I thought, "Why waste our time for just an excuse and not pay for the visit? Get it from the ER or ortho doctor."

A male presented with pain in the urethra. He thought he had an STD so he used a bulb syringe and pushed peroxide up his penis. I wanted to say, "You idiot, of course it is going to hurt if you put something up your urethra. You need to stop doing that and use condoms."

A patient stated she needed something for nasal congestion. "I haven't been able to breathe out of my nose forever." The entire time I was in there to examine her, she was breathing just fine out of her nose with her mouth closed. Just being here must have cured her. She was also obese and smoked, so I wanted to add, "Since you have food or cigarettes in your mouth the majority of the time, you have been able to breathe out of your mouth."

A patient came in complaining of discomfort with urination. We did a urinalysis, and I entered the room and stated, "Your urinalysis indicates that you have a bladder infection." I was shocked at the response from the patient. She said, "You're shittin' me. I knew that, and I don't even have a medical degree." I wanted to say, "Well then, tell me how to treat you too since you are so smart."

There are a lot of old wives' tales about poison ivy, but this one is very unusual. A patient stated he used gasoline on his skin to cure the poison ivy. The provider wanted to say, "If you had used a match too, it might have worked."

A patient had a superficial laceration. He stated, "It

feels like bone pain." I wanted to respond, "Oh, what does bone pain feel like? Didn't know there was a difference from regular pain."

This seventy-two-year-old came in stating that her gynecologist diagnosed her with vaginal yeast infection. She came into the clinic due to a sore throat and wanted to know if her boyfriend could have transmitted the yeast from her vagina to her mouth. Sometimes we heard more information than we needed to.

A mom brought in a child, and their hygiene was bad. The mother stated, "She came back from her dad's sick because they are dirty people." I wanted to ask, "Worse than you?"

A male came in concerned about an STD and stated, "I could have a STD because my ex- girlfriend was informed by a friend that a friend of his friend said the girl's ex-boyfriend has discharge from his penis. What is discharge?" I responded, "Anything draining from your dick." But I wanted to add, "And you need intelligence to have intercourse without condoms."

A patient came in complaining of something, but after examination and tests, we found nothing wrong with him. She agreed nothing was wrong but wanted us to sign a paper for the taxi so welfare would pay for it, and she wanted him to take her to the grocery store before going home. Isn't there something wrong with this picture?

A patient brought in medicine bottles of medication she

was given the last time she was sick and stated, "This helped so I want the same thing." I wanted to ask, "Do you mind if I examine you since you are paying for it? And then I'll decide based on my findings and knowledge if that is what you need. I'm so glad that all of us medical providers go to school for years just so patients can tell us what to prescribe."

Obesity is becoming a huge problem. We had a young patient come into the urgent care, and she was four feet tall and weighed 250 pounds. We wanted to ask if her nickname was "Refrigerator," but hopefully primary care providers are addressing these issues.

A patient came in complaining of pain from her knee that she had replaced years ago. She was wearing slacks. And she asked if I could tell she had a total knee. I wanted to say, "No, I can't see through clothing."

A male gentleman came in for complaints of a cold. He was serious and stated, "You can't tell if I have a cold by looking in my mouth because I had my tonsils removed." I had to think about it for a while and just said, "Okay, but I think I'll check your throat anyway." I wanted to say, "Okay, then bend over, and maybe if I check that end, I can tell."

Parents brought in a four-year-old, stating he had nausea, vomiting, and diarrhea. The symptoms presented for two days. They stated that they took him to lunch today and had to force him to eat half of a pizza, so they knew he was sick. I couldn't believe what I just heard, but I wanted to say, "You needed to make him eat the whole thing and chase it with some whiskey, and maybe he would be well by now."

A person came in for nausea, vomiting, and diarrhea for three hours. He wanted a work slip, and I offered him one for the next day because he had to go in at midnight. He said, "Oh, I need more time off than that." I wanted to say, "You're not really that ill, and if I have to work, so do you."

A three-year-old came in with his mother. She reported that he had been vomiting since yesterday. She asked him what sounded good to eat, and he said Taco Bell. So she took him to Taco Bell, and he ate and vomited again. She stated, "I don't know what to do." I wanted to reply, "You don't ask a three-year-old who is vomiting what he wants to eat any more than you ask him if he wants to play in the street or go to school." He was only three for God's sake. Who was the adult here, the one who should have had some common sense?

A patient came in after eating a pound of hot fries and complained of burning in his rectum and explosive diarrhea. I wanted to tell him, "Next time, put them in your butt, and maybe your mouth will burn."

Parents oftentimes just didn't take charge. A twelve-year-old came in and needed medication. She couldn't swallow pills, so the mother asked what flavor the medicine was. I said, "I don't know. Why?" The mother responded, "She won't take it if it is cherry flavored." Now this kid was twelve years old. I wanted to say, "If she needs it, then she needs to just take it."

Then there is the thought process that you have to have white patches on your tonsils to have strep throat or that you don't have strep throat because you don't have white patches on your tonsils. So patients came in with sore throats and said, "I don't have strep because I don't have white patches on my tonsils." I would have loved to say, "Oh, are yours purple or green?"

A sixteen-year-old female came in with her mother. The patient reported nausea and pain in the upper abdomen. I proceeded to examine the patient, and she was tender in the upper abdomen over her stomach. The mother spoke up and said, "She isn't nauseated, and she is tender in the pelvic region." I stood there and said to the mother, "Did you not see me just examine her abdomen? She said that it hurt when I pushed in her upper abdomen, not over her pelvic area?" The patient had told her mother that her stomach hurt, not her pelvis. I was sure the mother was not happy with my comment, but there was a time when a child was old enough to tell us what his or her symptoms were without the help of the parent.

A female patient reported that her clitoris was swollen and tender. I asked if she had oral sex, and she said, "Yes, frequently." I simply responded, "Give it a rest."

A mother brought in a child for ear infection. The child had already been treated with an antibiotic that was ordered three times a day, but the mother couldn't remember to give it three times a day. The ear was still infected, so I ordered a daily antibiotic so the mother could remember to give it to him. When I went to discharge them, the mother asked for a slip for the daycare to give him his once-a-day antibiotic. I just looked at the mother and asked, "Don't you see your child every day?" She said yes. I then replied, "Then I think you can be responsible to give it to him." Some people should just not be parents.

Patients asking for school and work excuses were a real problem. Parents kept kids home, and people didn't go to work when they had been sick for three days and wanted us to excuse them for the prior two days. We had no way of knowing if they were sick or not, but they got upset if we didn't do it. When your reimbursement was based on patient satisfaction, it put us in a position to do things we didn't like to do.

I had a grandmother bring in a child one late afternoon and requested a work slip for the child's mother who missed work because she stayed home with the child. Yet she didn't bring in the child. I gave her one but did comment that the mother should have brought her in.

Another example of that was a child who ran a fever for one hour one week ago and missed school, and the mother wanted an excuse for that day. The child was here and not ill. That one was refused.

A mother brought in a six-year-old due to vomiting

twice and diarrhea three times. She was concerned and wanted tests run to check for renal failure. When asked why, she responded because it ran in the family. Of course these relatives were in their late eighties. The provider wanted to say, "He could not eat for one week, and maybe his weight would come down to what it should be. And if he's in renal failure, it's too late to save him anyway." Obviously we didn't do unnecessary testing.

A grandmother brought in a five-month-old and said, "He has a sore throat." She didn't say he didn't want to eat or something significant. I wanted to respond, "Boy, if he can talk already, he is really advanced for his age."

A patient came in complaining of a sore wrist. He had fallen four months prior. I did ask, "Why did you wait so long?" But I wanted to say, "If you did break it, I'm not going to break it again to make it right because you were stupid and didn't come in." The sad thing was that he did break it, as seen on x-ray.

Maybe you have heard the old joke, "How many Pollocks does it take to change a light bulb?" The answer is one to hold the light bulb and six to move the ladder in a circle. Well, sometimes we wondered how many people were needed to bring in a patient. We had a great-grandmother, grandmother, and mother all in the room with a child. They all had their own ideas about what was wrong with the child. Even some adults would bring two to three people with them. It was like they had no better place to go to hang out.

Then sometimes a parent would bring in her child, and another adult was in the room as well. We asked the parent a question about the child, and the other person answered. We wanted to ask, "Who is the parent here?" There should be some type of test you have to pass to be a parent.

A grandmother brought in her granddaughter for cold symptoms. The grandmother said her doctor couldn't get her in, so she came to us. The grandmother stated, "Her doctor smells her skin to rule out a virus." I wanted to ask, "Why doesn't he lick her? It works better."

A patient came in for a possible bladder infection. I asked if she took baths, and she said no because her gynecologist said it would give her a vaginal infection. I think she got confused about a bladder infection versus vaginal. I thought, "Your vagina is already dirty, honey, but let's keep the bladder clean."

A mother brought in a child because she had a fever for three days. "I read on the Motrin bottle not to use for more than three days." I'm not sure if this is accurate, but most viral infections cause fevers for five days, so that is crazy.

Rashes were a very common complaint. Most dermatologists will teach you, if it is wet, dry it. If it is dry, wet it. If you don't want it, don't touch it!

A girl came in and wanted checked for chlamydia, an STD. She stated her ex-boyfriend called her, and he was positive. Her new boyfriend came in with her. He asked me to treat her with the antibiotic today so he didn't have to wait for the results to be able to screw her without condoms. It took two days for the results. He responded, "Two days! Really." I thought, "This isn't about you, and if you don't want her to give you something, masturbate."

Patients were really rude. They were also coming in two to three minutes before we closed. Our sign saying "open" could even be turned off, but we couldn't lock the door because patients were still in the building to leave. Usually they had been sick two days but couldn't wait. We saw them but would have loved to say, "Sorry, we are closed. Why didn't you come in a lot earlier if you've been sick for two days?" I don't go into any store or establishment now if they getting ready to close. It's just rude.

A patient came in for a workman's compensation claim. She said she wouldn't pass the required drug screen. I asked why, and she said, "Because my boyfriend takes heroin and I swallow when I suck on him." How do you respond to that? I just said, "Well, we are going to do it anyway."

A parent brought in a baby for nasal congestion. We instructed her on how to use baby nose drops and the bulb syringe to suck out his nose. She said, "I know how to do that, but he doesn't like it, so I don't do it." I thought, "For goodness sakes, he wasn't going to like it when he has to go to school someday or do his homework. But who is the parent? Do it anyway!"

A man came in because of blood in his urine. He said, "My wife and I had sex, and she was on her period." I thought, "Sorry, but it doesn't travel up to your bladder that way."

A woman said she got a vaginal infection because her husband refused to go pee after they had intercourse. I thought, "No, you get a bladder infection when you don't go pee after intercourse." I swear that people get everything confused what we try to teach them.

A husband and wife came in and were both positive for chlamydia and gonorrhea. The wife also had bacterial vaginosis, which is not a STD. She said, "I can't believe this infection can be that bad to cause us to get chlamydia and GC." I looked at her and wanted to say, "You bitch, you cheated and don't want to admit it."

An elderly lady came in demanding a shot for her cold. I told her it wasn't indicated. And she said, "Okay then, I'll just die." Good luck with that one. I wanted to say, "You are eighty-three, so I guess you've lived long enough." I gave her a prescription for oral medicine, and she left very upset.

When guys came in for testing for STDs, some nationalities took pride in the size of their penis. Well, I guess most guys do. I would have loved to say, "Well, it looks like a penis, just smaller."

Others came in and said, "I have a cough, and when I cough, I wet myself." I wanted to say, "Well, wear dark clothes. It will make you feel nice and warm, and no one will notice."

Other people came in and said, "I have nausea, and I

vomited for one day, which was yesterday. I need a work excuse for today." I wanted to say, "Eating too much kimchi can do that to you. Go to work."

On work physical forms, they asked for the color of eyes and hair. I asked a child once what color his eyes were. He responded, "Brown, but if you are color-blind, don't they change colors?" I wanted to say, "No, that isn't what that means." But I was thinking, "You got to be kidding me."

A woman came in thinking she had head lice and maybe scabies. She recently had her doctors remove an old tampon that she forgot was in her vagina for weeks. So now she thought she also had toxic shock syndrome because, when she walked by someone, she shocked him or her. I wanted to say, "It's not an electrical problem, you idiot."

A man had poison ivy on his arm. He thought bleach would treat it. So he didn't just wipe off his arm with bleach water. He soaked his arm in straight bleach. He had a nasty chemical burn. I wanted to ask, "Why didn't you consult someone first? What the hell were you thinking?"

A lady came in complaining of loss of bladder control and tingling and numbness in arms and legs. "The problems started when the tenant living below me started playing his music so loud that it makes my bed shake." I thought, "Then you should ask him to turn it down or sleep in your bathtub."

People love to "pop" pimples. A mother brought in her five-month-old son. She thought she saw a pimple on his scrotum so she tried to pop it. His entire scrotum on the left side was red and infected. If you ever see a red area on your baby, have it checked, or try soap and water. But don't mess with it. Poor, defenseless child.

A patient was complaining of sweaty feet, so he used alcohol and was now complaining of dry skin. I advised some lotion, but next time, he was to sit in the sun for his sweaty feet with nothing on them and drink the alcohol instead.

There were also various reasons why people needed refills on medication. Pharmacists even reported to me some of these popular reasons, especially for controlled meds and antibiotics:

- "I was opening my Xanax bottle over the fish aquarium, and my pills fell in."
- "I put my meds on the back of my motorcycle, and they fell off."
- "My son flushed them down the toilet."
- "We moved, and I must have packed them somewhere and can't find them."
- "I stayed overnight in another town and left them there."
- "I thought I was having a side effect, so I pitched them, but I realized it wasn't. So I need some more."

Some people's pain threshold was very low. A male patient stubbed his toe. There was no bruising or swelling. No fracture was seen on x-ray. He demanded crutches because he couldn't walk on it. I wanted to say, "No, but I'll refer you to a urologist for a testicle implant."

Someone reported a problem with nausea in mornings if awakened with an alarm clock. If the alarm clock didn't work and he slept in, he was okay. I wanted to say, "Go to bed earlier on the days you work. No time off. Sorry, buddy."

Another patient said he needed Xanax to sleep; otherwise he would drink two vodkas to sleep. I wanted to say, "Enjoy your vodka."

Another patient said, "I need some Tramadol. I know it isn't a narcotic because it doesn't mess up my head." I thought, "So I guess drugs have to make you feel high to be addicting. Gee, I didn't know that. By the way, it is on the narcotics list of controlled substances."

One patient came in for a sore throat and was given Magic Mouthwash, a mixture of Maalox, viscous lidocaine, and Benadryl. She wanted to know if she could snuff it to help with her nose. She was five months pregnant. I thought, "No, that is why they call it a mouthwash. I don't really care, but it won't give you the effect you maybe get from your cocaine. Maybe snorting an antibiotic would help, but you don't need one for a viral infection." That poor baby didn't stand a chance.

A patient reported with conjunctivitis, or "pink eye." I told him not to wear his contacts until he saw well. If he did, he could harm his cornea and cause problems with his vision for life. He said, "Well, I have to see, and my glasses don't work." I thought, "Okay, chose short-term vision problems for your entire lifetime." Sometimes I thought I was talking to a teenager and not a grown adult.

There were people who abused the system. A patient was seen for another problem, but it was noticed that he was on Medicare for a disability, alcoholism. So he was getting paid for a self-induced problem. And guess what? He was still drinking. There was no accountability. What is wrong with this picture?

A woman was expecting her third child. She was not married, and her mother had custody of the first child. She was on welfare for psychiatric problems and got more money every month if she had another child. How do we stop this?

There were a few comments when I couldn't think of a good response. A woman asked if she could get pregnant from her dog. Then another one inquired if she could get an STD from a dog. I simply responded, "No."

I had a farmer who had to catheterize himself due to obstructive problems. He would stick the catheter in his farm hat, and when he had to use it, he would get it out and stick it in his mouth to lubricate it. And after he had catheterized himself, he put it back in his hat for the next time. He never got an infection. Well, so much for sanitization.

A patient had amoxicillin listed under her allergies. The side effect was, "It just doesn't work." I explained to her that that it was not an allergy. She probably had a cold, and that was why it didn't work. Antibiotics won't get you better if you have a virus.

A lady came in stating she was diagnosed with cysts. One ruptured, but the other ended up being a baby. I said most cysts were on the ovaries. I asked, "Was this inside your uterus?" She responded yes. I thought, "Sorry, a cyst doesn't turn into a baby. Once a baby, always a baby."

A patient was seen for an insect bite on his thumb. "I can't go back to work, right?" I thought, "Wrong! You are going back since we have to pay for your Benadryl that you should be buying over the counter and not getting free since you are on Medicaid."

Another patient said, "Veins are burning in my arms and legs. I think I have some kind of toxin in me." The patient was referred to psychiatrist. I thought, "Your veins are fine, but your head isn't."

A patient came in having shoulder pain for two years and had an appointment to see an orthopedic doctor in four days. I thought, "You can wait two years but can't wait four more days!"

A seven-year-old girl came in and was diagnosed with a canker sore. I told her mother I could give her something for the soreness, but I couldn't cure it. The girl looked at me and said, "I want it gone *now*." I was so shocked that I just walked out. The mother never said a word to correct her.

A patient came here from out of town and stated that the ATM machine ate her credit card. She asked if her prescription would be free. I thought, "No! Not everything is free. Machines don't just eat cards for no reason."

One patient was seen in the ER for constipation and given MaltSupax. He started to have a bowel movement after two days. But he kept taking it and was now here for diarrhea. I thought, "Stop taking the medicine, you idiot."

A patient came in complaining of fatigue. In questioning him, he had been deer hunting. Then he went to work and slept for two hours. I thought, "Go home and sleep! Would you waste your money to come in for something like this?"

One patient said the car door closed on her two fingers six days ago. She worked at McDonald's, and her fingers were hurt and tingly. Her hands were dirty, and when I entered the room, she held up a finger to have me wait a minute because she was on the phone. She told the person on the phone that she had just finished changing the tire herself. She came in for a sore hand yet had just changed a tire. It was obviously not that sore. I thought, "Also don't tell me to wait. I have better things to do and other patients to see." I should've left and kept her waiting. Obviously she wanted a note for work. She couldn't work at McDonald's but could change a tire.

A child came in with his dad. She was thirteen and didn't go to school because Dad couldn't get her out of bed. She was not sick. She just didn't want to go to school. She didn't need to learn anymore, according to the girl. She could get a job and make two hundred dollars a year, and that was okay. She just wanted a note for missing school. She and the father were sent for counseling. We couldn't excuse teenager's behavior. I couldn't believe why some people came to an urgent care.

One of our nurses asked a patient if she took anything for a fever. She replied, "Yes, I took Benadryl." The nurse thought, "Boy, must be a new indication!"

A patient came in stating that he sprained his foot and it hurt on the bottom. He said, "I think my arch fell." I thought, "It's not something that falls, but pick it up and tie it back on."

A patient stated, "I have nausea, vomiting, and diarrhea." When asked how long, he said, "For as long as I can remember." He was twenty-eight years old.

A patient reported that drinking a lot of pop caused him to get sinus congestion and increased sinus pressure. I thought, "Well, stop drinking pop!"

A lady looked up wait time at our facility on the computer, and it was two hours. So she showed up two hours later, thinking she'd get right in.

A patient reported, "I get bladder infections with the change in seasons." I thought, "Then move to an area where the seasons don't change that much."

A patient had COPD and smoked. He had bronchitis, so I asked if he were using his aerosol machine. He said, "I can't because I broke my right hand." I thought, "Then how do you light your cigarettes?"

An eighty-nine-year-old woman said she had electricity from her hand, and when she touched her neck, it made her neck hurt. I thought, "If your hand produces electricity, can you turn on a lamp by holding the chord?"

A grandmother brought in her granddaughter with her. She had been diagnosed with a UTI. Before they left, she told her granddaughter, "Don't drink after me, or you will get my UTI." I just looked at her and thought, "I didn't just hear that, did I?"

A patient came in complaining that the prescribed eye drops were draining down her throat and making her cough. I thought, "Where in the hell are you putting the eye drops?"

One patient complained, "I know I have a sinus infection because my pipes are burning." I thought, "Your what are burning?"

I told a mother that she had to rinse her eight-year-old's ears with warm water weekly for wax removal. The mother looked at the eight-year-old and asked, "Honey, will you let me do that?" I thought, "When do you ask an eight-year-old for permission to do something that is necessary? Instead she'd rather pay the bill for us to do it, and we don't ask permission."

There was this perfectly normal fourteen-year-old boy, and his mother said to him in front of me, "Do you have to go potty before we leave?" Really, how embarrassing.

A patient was diagnosed with ringworm and had a cat. The patient asked, "The cat scratches me, and I lick it. Could I have gotten it that way?"

The woman reported that her husband cheated on her. The mistress called her and reported she was positive for chlamydia, so the patient wanted tested. She also wanted to know if her child could get it because she was breastfeeding. I thought, "I've never heard of STDs being obtained through breast milk, but is your child sexually active?" I think she had a bigger problem to be concerned about.

A patient called, unhappy he had been given a steroid for his sore throat from a virus to help with the swelling. He commented that it was like being given a shotgun to kill a mosquito. I wanted to tell him, "If you are upset, come back, and we will give you a fly swatter."

A patient stated his stools were black from taking Tylenol. I thought, "No, but it is from the Pepto-Bismol you are taking."

A guy came in concerned because he had his drink sitting for a while, and when he started to drink it again, he saw a dead mouse in it as he was drinking. He was concerned about getting something from the mouse. I'd worry more about whatever killed the mouse. Boy, what an athletic mouse to get in there without spilling the cup!

A mother brought in a toddler after finding him chewing on an old used condom. She wanted to be sure he couldn't get anything from it. I thought, "Well, at least we don't have to worry about him getting pregnant."

A patient stated he coughed so hard that he busted his "calapitories." He meant his capillaries.

A patient stated that he took Benadryl and wondered why it didn't take his fever down. I don't think it is a fever medicine. I thought, "Maybe keep it for if you have an allergic reaction to something!"

Patient reported she had a rash because she had deleted pop from her diet. I thought, "You can't go cold turkey. Try weaning slower."

A patient was allergic to several antibiotics, so her doctor gave her a steroid every time she was prescribed a new antibiotic so she didn't have a reaction to it. She insisted I give her a steroid with the antibiotic I gave her, which wasn't on her allergy list. I thought, "I hope you never develop an allergy to the steroids!"

A patient said, "I know my ears are healthy. That's why I produce so much wax." I thought, "Did you breastfeed? I bet your breasts would have produced a lot of milk too."

A person recording the patient's complaint put down that he had diarrhea. When the provider entered the room and said, "I understand you have diarrhea," the patient said, "No, I have gonorrhea." It's a good thing it wasn't the other way around.

A patient stated he was "going blind from pain." I thought, "Watch your hearing. It may go next."

A boy was brought in with nausea and vomiting. He was caught licking a cat that came out from the sewer. I wouldn't have said anything because the poor child had some mental development delays, but what a case.

A patient once told the provider that she couldn't use any nasal sprays because they made her have a fever. I thought, "What do cough syrups do?"

A patient said, "When I take deep breaths, it pushes oxygen into my eye, and they water." I thought, "When you cough, do they dry up?"

A patient was in the hospital and had a chest tube several weeks before. The patient said, "The lungs are fine, but the fluid and air that was in my lung moved to my bowels, and now I'm gassy." I thought, "Sorry, but there's no direct path from the lungs to your gut."

A child came in due to a red eye. I asked if his eye hurt, and he said yes because his brother farted in his face.

A patient reported that his fever was 108 degrees the night before. I thought, "Did smoke come out of your ears or nose?"

Compazine was listed as an allergy. It causes increased body odor. A patient stated she was allergic to Stadol. It made her go into labor even when not pregnant. Really? One patient even stated he had fifteen side effects to a drug by reading the information given with it. I thought, "Don't read the information."

Tattoos are sometime entertaining. A patient came in for STD testing. During the pelvic exam, the provider noticed a tattoo in her pubic region that said "Lucky." If she were positive for anything, the guy wasn't that lucky.

Many patients came in when they had only been sick

for twenty-four hours. We would have loved to say, "Oh my, why did you wait so long? If you would have come in sooner, I might have been able to save you."

A patient came in because of tooth pain and stated he didn't brush his teeth because they were decayed already. I wanted to ask, "Why bother to wipe your ass because it's only going to get dirty again?"

We asked patients for a stool specimen, and he urinated in the cup. He was told, "No, we need some poop."

I told a patient, "You got an infection." He asked, "What does that mean?" I repeated, "You have a bacterial infection." Again he said, "What does that mean?" I said, "You have a bug." He responded, "Oh no! I have bugs!" I couldn't win.

A patient reported that her arm, head, and legs were flying all over. We sent her to the ER because she thought she was having a seizure. The ER doctor asked if we were sending her by ambulance, and the provider replied, "I never have heard of a patient having a grand mal seizure and remembering the details of it. No, she is flying over." He didn't want to deal with her.

A patient came in stating ear drops that her doctor had prescribed was causing her eyes to drain and made her cough and have hot flashes. I thought, "Are you putting the drops in other places by mistake?"

A wife had a yeast infection, and I explained to the couple that it was not contagious or transmitted by intercourse. The husband stated, "Well in the olden days, it was because I got it really bad from my girlfriend." I only said, "Well, maybe back then, but not now."

A woman came in with her daughter and granddaughter, complaining of a cough. She was concerned she had pneumonia. The lungs sounded fine, but I got a chest x-ray, and it was normal. After I told her it was just a viral infection, she said she was certain she had it because her grandmother was just diagnosed with it. I told them that you really can't get pneumonia from someone else unless you handle the person's mucous and don't wash your hands or maybe intimately kiss him or her. The patient's grandmother stated the baby, who was a year old, had coughed up phlegm and spit it into her mouth. So she knew she had it because she now had it. Obviously I refused to give her an antibiotic and wanted to say, "Well, you should have just spit it back into her mouth, and you would be okay."

A man came in complaining that, when he tapped his balls together, the veins in them hurt. I thought, "Why are you tapping your balls together anyway? Stop doing that. They aren't ping-pong balls!"

We didn't always get the truth. A patient stated she went to the ER for a sore throat and was given a laxative. I checked the ER report. Her complaint was abdominal pain, and she was constipated. Yet it was the ER provider's fault that she had a sore throat and missed work.

A patient complained that his ejaculation was too thick.

I wanted to tell him to let it rest. He was to increase his water intake, and if that didn't work, he could douche with vinegar.

A patient came in for a cough. He went home, took one dose of medication, and then called back, stating she was still coughing. I wanted to say that we couldn't do anything more and she would probably die by morning.

An allergic reaction was explained as an "out-of-body experience." I thought, "That's unusual. Most people pay extra for that."

A mother asked if a child could still be teething after he has all his teeth. I thought, "What do you think teething means?"

I was explaining that Tessalon Perles were a cough suppressant. The patient stated, "Like a cough drop?" I thought, "You got it. Just more expensive."

A patient complained of nausea and abdominal pain for one month. "My piercing of the belly button is causing it." I thought, "Your belly button isn't connected to the nausea center in your brain."

A patient said, "I might have bronchitis or a UTI because my vagina hurts with my periods." I thought, "Maybe your vagina has bronchitis. Maybe we could insert an antibiotic into your vagina and see if it works."

A patient was seen for a sport injury. There was a free clinic for follow-up for sport injuries. The patient complained that it was too early in the morning to go. I thought, "Then maybe you can find another free one that sees patients later in the day so you can sleep in. What do you want for *free*?"

A patient was seen for a STD but didn't get his medication. He returned to the clinic and wanted it for free. I thought, "Sorry, we don't pay for bad ill responsible behavior."

A patient came in complaining of stomach pains for three days, saying it hurt to eat. After examining her, we discussed the problem and diet. She said, "You mean I can't eat pizza tonight?" I thought, "Are you an idiot? What did I just say?"

A patient asked if a vaginal yeast infection came from masturbating. The provider said, "Gee, I hope not." One really strange complaint was, "My stomach feels other people's madness and sadness for the last five years."

A patient named Rikki complained of rash on wrist and genitals. We figured it was a guy and was poison ivy from peeing in the woods. I walked into the room, and it was a girl, not a guy. But it was poison ivy from peeing in the woods. Can't be gender bias.

Printed in the United States
By Bookmasters